Navigating Life with Crohn's Disease

A Comprehensive Guide to Understanding, Managing, and Thriving with Inflammatory Bowel Disease

Dr. Oftelith S.

Copyright©2024 Dr. Oftelith S.

All rights reserved.

Disclaimer

The information provided in this book is intended for personal and educational purposes only. It is not a substitute for professional medical advice, diagnosis, or treatment. Readers are urged to consult healthcare professionals for personalized guidance. The author and publisher disclaim any responsibility for adverse effects resulting from the information. Individuals diagnosed with one problem or another are advised to undergo regular medical check-ups and consult with healthcare experts for ongoing monitoring and necessary advice. The contents of this book are not for sale or public use without explicit permission, emphasizing the importance of respecting intellectual property rights.

Table of Contents

INTRODUCTION 3
   Overview 6
   What do you understand by Crohn's Disease 7
SYMPTOMS 8
CAUSES 12
RISK FACTORS AND COMPLICATIONS OF CROHN'S DISEASE 17
   Risk Factors 17
   Complications 19
DIAGNOSIS 22
TREATMENT AND MEDICATIONS 26
CONCLUSION 32
Appendix 33
   Dietary Considerations 33
   Carefully Selected Food Diet 37
   Some Key Facts About Crohn's Disease 77
   Medical Advice and Tips 79
Glossary of Terms 82

INTRODUCTION

Life is incredibly fulfilling when you are active and able to move around freely. Now, imagine facing a health challenge that has no cure—I'm sure that's quite unsettling. This is the reality for many individuals battling diseases like Crohn's, which currently have no cure. However, it can be managed with treatments that prevent flare-ups and control symptoms. As I always emphasize, health is paramount, and vigilance is key to maintaining well-being. Before we delve further, I urge you to prioritize self-care, for a healthy life is a life well lived.

This book explores Crohn's disease, a condition without a definitive cure. Nonetheless, numerous therapies provide hope by managing symptoms and fostering long-term relief from inflammation.

But what if we could prevent it altogether? Prevention, after all, is the cornerstone of vitality.

If you haven't been diagnosed with Crohn's, consider yourself fortunate. Preparation is crucial. And if you have been diagnosed, don't worry. You'll learn to navigate daily challenges with adjustments and therapies that promote longevity.

Every page of this book contains invaluable insights. By the end of your journey, you'll understand the intricacies of Crohn's disease—its symptoms, causes, risk factors, complications, and effective management strategies.

Take a moment to gather yourself; we're about to embark on an enlightening exploration. Ready? Let's dive in!

Overview

This book offers essential guidance for individuals navigating the complexities of Crohn's disease, a chronic condition impacting the digestive tract. This comprehensive resource provides insights into the symptoms, causes, and management strategies of Crohn's disease, empowering readers to make informed decisions about their health. Whether you're living with Crohn's disease, caring for someone who is, or simply seeking to broaden your understanding of this condition, this book is for you. It emphasizes proactive self-care, lifestyle adjustments, and preventive measures as key components of promoting overall well-being, making it a valuable resource for everyone, regardless of their health status.

What do you understand by Crohn's Disease

Crohn's disease is a chronic inflammatory bowel disease (IBD) characterized by inflammation of the digestive tract. This condition can affect any part of the gastrointestinal tract, from the mouth to the anus, but it most commonly involves the small intestine and the beginning of the large intestine (colon). Crohn's disease is characterized by periods of flare-ups, during which symptoms worsen, followed by periods of remission. Symptoms may include abdominal pain, diarrhea, fatigue, weight loss, and malnutrition. Crohn's disease is a lifelong condition with no known cure, but various treatment options are available to manage symptoms and improve quality of life.

SYMPTOMS

Symptoms of Crohn's disease, a subset of inflammatory bowel diseases (IBDs), manifest in diverse ways, reflecting the complexity of this chronic condition:

- **Ileocolitis:** This prevalent form of Crohn's disease induces inflammation at the junction of the small intestine's final segment, known as the ileum, and the adjacent colon.

Signs to Watch for: Keep an eye out for significant weight fluctuations, persistent diarrhea, abdominal cramps, and localized discomfort, typically concentrated in the mid to lower right abdomen.

- **Ileitis:** Focused solely on the ileum, this variant brings inflammation to the small intestine's concluding portion.

Signs to Watch for: Expect similar indicators to ileocolitis, including weight fluctuations, diarrhea, abdominal cramps, and localized discomfort in the middle to lower right abdomen. Additionally, be vigilant for the potential development of fistulas or inflammatory abscesses in the lower right abdominal region.

- **Gastroduodenal Crohn's Disease**: This unique subtype impacts both the stomach and the initial segment of the small intestine, known as the duodenum.

Indications to Observe: Watch for nausea, noticeable weight changes, decreased appetite, and vomiting, especially if segments of the bowel become obstructed.

- **Jejunoileitis**: Characterized by inflammation in the jejunum, the middle section of the small intestine.

Recognizable Signs: Look out for cramping sensations post-meals, the potential formation of fistulas, diarrhea, and escalating abdominal discomfort.

- **Crohn's (Granulomatous) Colitis:** This particular variant focuses solely on the colon.

Symptoms to Monitor: Keep an eye out for skin abnormalities, joint discomfort, diarrhea, rectal bleeding, and the emergence of ulcers, fistulas, and abscesses around the anus.

It's important to acknowledge that symptomatology may overlap between these types, with multiple regions of the digestive tract simultaneously affected. Additionally, Crohn's disease can be further classified based on phenotypic characteristics, which include the age at diagnosis and specific traits related to the disease's behavior and affected body parts. These traits encompass stricturing, penetrating, and uncomplicated phenotypes.

CAUSES

Crohn's disease is a multifactorial condition characterized by chronic inflammation of the gastrointestinal tract. While the precise etiology of Crohn's disease remains incompletely understood, several factors are believed to contribute to its development:

- **Immune System Dysfunction:**

    - A prevailing hypothesis suggests that Crohn's disease results from an aberrant immune response in genetically susceptible individuals. In this scenario, the body's immune system mistakenly identifies harmless substances, such as food particles or intestinal bacteria, as foreign invaders and launches an inflammatory response.

    - This chronic inflammation leads to tissue damage and ulceration within the digestive tract, resulting in the characteristic symptoms of Crohn's disease, such as abdominal pain, diarrhea, and weight loss.

- **Genetic Predisposition:**

  - Genetic factors play a significant role in the susceptibility to Crohn's disease. Individuals with a family history of the condition are at an increased risk of developing it themselves, highlighting the hereditary component of the disease.

  - While specific genetic mutations associated with Crohn's disease have been identified, such as variants in genes related to immune function and barrier integrity in the gut, the precise genetic architecture of the disease remains complex and heterogeneous.

- **Environmental Triggers:**

- Environmental factors are thought to play a crucial role in triggering the onset of Crohn's disease or exacerbating existing symptoms in genetically susceptible individuals.

- Potential environmental triggers include diet, particularly high-fat and low-fiber diets, smoking, microbial infections, exposure to certain medications (such as nonsteroidal anti-inflammatory drugs), and environmental pollutants.

- These environmental factors can disrupt the delicate balance of the gut microbiota, leading to dysbiosis and dysregulation of immune responses within the intestinal mucosa.

- **Microbial Dysbiosis:**

- Alterations in the composition and function of the gut microbiota, known as dysbiosis, have been implicated in the pathogenesis of Crohn's disease.

- Dysbiosis can result from factors such as antibiotic use, dietary changes, and environmental exposures, leading to imbalances in beneficial and harmful bacteria within the gut.

- These microbial imbalances can trigger inflammatory responses and contribute to the perpetuation of chronic intestinal inflammation in individuals with Crohn's disease.

- **Epigenetic Modifications:**

    - Epigenetic changes, which involve alterations in gene expression without changes to the underlying DNA sequence, may also contribute to the development of Crohn's disease.

- Environmental factors such as diet, stress, and exposure to toxins can induce epigenetic modifications that influence immune function and inflammatory responses in the gut.

- These epigenetic changes may contribute to the dysregulation of immune responses and the perpetuation of chronic inflammation in individuals predisposed to Crohn's disease.

RISK FACTORS AND COMPLICATIONS OF CROHN'S DISEASE

Crohn's disease is a complex condition influenced by various risk factors, and it can lead to several complications that significantly impact an individual's quality of life. Understanding these risk factors and complications is crucial for disease management and prevention.

Risk Factors

- **Genetics:** Family history plays a significant role in the development of Crohn's disease. Individuals with a first-degree relative, such as a parent, sibling, or child, with Crohn's disease have a higher risk of developing the condition themselves.

- **Age:** While Crohn's disease can occur at any age, it most commonly develops in adolescents and young adults. However, a growing number of cases are being diagnosed in older adults.

- **Ethnicity:** Crohn's disease affects people of all ethnicities, but certain populations, such as individuals of Ashkenazi Jewish descent and those of European ancestry, have a higher risk.

- **Smoking:** Cigarette smoking is a significant modifiable risk factor for Crohn's disease. Smokers have a higher risk of developing the condition compared to nonsmokers, and smoking can also worsen disease severity and increase the risk of complications.

- **Nonsteroidal Anti-Inflammatory Drugs (NSAIDs):** Long-term use of NSAIDs, such as ibuprofen and naproxen, may increase the risk of developing Crohn's disease or exacerbate existing symptoms in susceptible individuals.

Complications
- **Bowel Obstruction:** Chronic inflammation and scarring of the intestinal walls can lead to the formation of strictures, or narrowed areas, causing bowel obstruction. This can result in abdominal pain, bloating, vomiting, and constipation.

- **Ulcers and Fistulas:** Inflammation within the digestive tract can lead to the formation of ulcers, open sores that may bleed and cause pain. Fistulas, abnormal connections between different parts of the intestine or between the intestine and other organs, can also develop, leading to complications such as abscesses and infections.

- **Malnutrition:** Chronic inflammation and impaired absorption of nutrients in the intestines can lead to malnutrition, resulting in weight loss, fatigue, weakness, and deficiencies in essential vitamins and minerals.

- **Perianal Complications:** Crohn's disease can affect the area around the anus, leading to complications such as anal fissures (tears in the tissue lining the anus), abscesses, and fistulas. These conditions can cause pain, discomfort, and difficulty with bowel movements.

- **Increased Risk of Colon Cancer:** Individuals with Crohn's disease affecting the colon have an increased risk of developing colorectal cancer, especially if the disease is long-standing or involves extensive inflammation. Regular colonoscopies are recommended for early detection and management of precancerous changes.

- **Extraintestinal Manifestations:** Crohn's disease can affect other organs and systems in the body, leading to extraintestinal complications such as arthritis, skin disorders, eye inflammation, liver disease, and osteoporosis.

DIAGNOSIS

Diagnosing Crohn's disease involves a comprehensive evaluation of the patient's medical history, symptoms, physical examination findings, and various diagnostic tests. Due to the nonspecific nature of Crohn's symptoms and the absence of a single definitive test, diagnosis often requires a multidisciplinary approach and careful consideration of clinical and laboratory findings.

Medical History and Physical Examination

- **Medical History:** The healthcare provider will inquire about the patient's symptoms, including abdominal pain, diarrhea, weight loss, fatigue, and other associated complaints. A detailed medical history, including any family history of inflammatory bowel disease (IBD), is essential in identifying potential risk factors.

- **Physical Examination:** A thorough physical examination may reveal signs such as abdominal tenderness, palpable masses, perianal disease (e.g., fistulas, abscesses), or extraintestinal manifestations (e.g., joint swelling, skin lesions).

Laboratory Tests

- **Blood Tests:** Blood tests may be conducted to assess inflammatory markers such as C-reactive protein (CRP) and erythrocyte sedimentation rate (ESR), which can indicate ongoing inflammation in the body. Additionally, blood tests may help identify anemia, nutritional deficiencies, and other abnormalities.

- **Stool Studies:** Stool samples may be analyzed for the presence of occult blood, infectious pathogens, or inflammatory markers, which can help differentiate Crohn's disease from other gastrointestinal conditions.

Imaging Studies

- **Endoscopy and Colonoscopy:** These procedures involve the insertion of a flexible, lighted tube equipped with a camera (endoscope) into the gastrointestinal tract to visualize the lining of the esophagus, stomach, small intestine, and colon. Biopsy samples may be obtained during these procedures to confirm the presence of inflammation and assess for characteristic features of Crohn's disease, such as granulomas.

- **Capsule Endoscopy:** In capsule endoscopy, the patient swallows a small, pill-sized camera that captures images as it passes through the digestive tract, providing a detailed view of the small intestine, where Crohn's disease commonly affects.

- **Imaging Studies:** Various imaging modalities, such as computed tomography (CT), magnetic resonance imaging (MRI), and ultrasound, may be used to evaluate the extent and severity of bowel inflammation, identify complications (e.g., strictures, fistulas, abscesses), and monitor disease progression over time.

- **Differential Diagnosis**

Given the overlapping symptoms and nonspecific nature of Crohn's disease, healthcare providers must consider alternative diagnoses, such as ulcerative colitis, infectious gastroenteritis, irritable bowel syndrome (IBS), celiac disease, and gastrointestinal malignancies. Additional diagnostic tests and consultation with gastroenterologists and other specialists may be necessary to rule out other conditions and confirm the diagnosis of Crohn's disease.

TREATMENT AND MEDICATIONS

Crohn's disease management aims to reduce inflammation, alleviate symptoms, achieve and maintain remission, and prevent complications. Treatment approaches vary based on disease severity, location, and patient response. A multidisciplinary approach involving healthcare providers, including gastroenterologists, nutritionists, and pharmacists, is essential to develop individualized treatment plans. Below are the primary treatment modalities and medications used in Crohn's disease management:

Anti-inflammatory Medications

- **Corticosteroids:** Prednisone and budesonide are commonly used to reduce inflammation and induce remission during flare-ups. However, long-term use is limited due to adverse effects such as bone loss, weight gain, and immunosuppression.

- **5-Aminosalicylates (5-ASAs):** While not as effective in Crohn's disease as in ulcerative colitis, 5-ASAs like sulfasalazine and mesalamine may help control mild to moderate inflammation, particularly in colonic involvement.

Immunosuppressive Agents

- **Azathioprine and Mercaptopurine:** These immunosuppressants are used as steroid-sparing agents to maintain remission and prevent relapses in moderate to severe Crohn's disease. Regular monitoring for side effects, including bone marrow suppression and liver toxicity, is essential.

- **Methotrexate:** Methotrexate may be prescribed for patients intolerant or refractory to other medications. It inhibits immune cell proliferation and reduces inflammation, but close monitoring for adverse effects such as hepatotoxicity and myelosuppression is necessary.

Biologic Therapies

- **Anti-Tumor Necrosis Factor (TNF) Agents:** Infliximab, adalimumab, and certolizumab pegol target TNF-alpha, a pro-inflammatory cytokine involved in Crohn's pathogenesis. These biologics are effective in inducing and maintaining remission, especially in patients with moderate to severe disease or those refractory to conventional therapies.

- **Anti-Integrin Therapy:** Vedolizumab selectively blocks leukocyte trafficking to the gut by inhibiting $\alpha 4\beta 7$ integrin, offering an alternative treatment option for patients intolerant or non-responsive to anti-TNF agents.

- **Anti-Interleukin (IL) Therapies:** Ustekinumab and risankizumab target IL-12/23 pathways, modulating immune responses and reducing inflammation. These biologics may be considered in patients with inadequate response to anti-TNF therapy.

Antibiotics

- **Metronidazole and Ciprofloxacin:** Antibiotics like metronidazole and ciprofloxacin may be used to treat perianal disease, fistulas, or abscesses associated with Crohn's disease. They can also help reduce bacterial overgrowth and mucosal inflammation.

Symptomatic Treatment

- **Anti-diarrheal Agents:** Loperamide may be used to control diarrhea and improve stool consistency, although caution is advised in patients with strictures or obstruction.

- **Pain Management:** Acetaminophen is recommended for mild to moderate pain relief in Crohn's disease, while opioids should be avoided due to their potential for exacerbating symptoms and dependency.

Nutritional Therapy

- **Enteral Nutrition:** Exclusive enteral nutrition (EEN) or partial enteral nutrition (PEN) may be recommended to induce remission in active Crohn's disease, particularly in children or patients with extensive small bowel involvement. Enteral feeding can improve nutritional status, promote mucosal healing, and reduce inflammation.

Surgery

- **Resection and Strictureplasty:** Surgical intervention may be necessary in patients with complications such as strictures, fistulas, abscesses, or refractory disease. Bowel resection and strictureplasty aim to remove diseased segments and alleviate obstructive symptoms while preserving bowel function.

CONCLUSION

If you have read through this book, Crohn's disease should no longer be a mystery to you. As promised, I hope it has provided valuable insights and enlightenment. For those diagnosed with Crohn's, there is no need for fear. Instead, focus on the necessary measures to manage the condition effectively. Always prioritize your health, as there is nothing more valuable than a healthy life. When you take care of your well-being, everything else will fall into place. Remember, a proactive approach to managing Crohn's disease can lead to a fulfilling and vibrant life.

Appendix

Dietary Considerations

1. **Low-Residue Diet:** A low-residue diet can help reduce bowel movements and minimize irritation to the gastrointestinal tract. This diet emphasizes consuming foods that are low in fiber and easily digestible, such as:

   - Refined grains (white bread, white rice)
   - Cooked fruits and vegetables without skins or seeds (applesauce, peeled potatoes)
   - Lean proteins (chicken, fish, eggs)
   - Dairy alternatives (lactose-free milk, yogurt)
   - Smooth nut butters (peanut butter, almond butter)

2. **Hydration:** Staying hydrated is crucial, especially during flare-ups or when taking

medications like corticosteroids that can increase the risk of dehydration. Choose water and electrolyte-rich beverages, such as:

- Plain water
- Coconut water
- Electrolyte drinks (Pedialyte)
- Herbal teas (chamomile, ginger)

3. **Probiotic-Rich Foods:** Probiotics may help promote gut health and balance the intestinal microbiota, potentially reducing inflammation and improving symptoms. Include probiotic-rich foods in your diet, such as:

- Yogurt with live active cultures
- Kefir
- Fermented vegetables (sauerkraut, kimchi)
- Tempeh

4. **Omega-3 Fatty Acids:** Omega-3 fatty acids have anti-inflammatory properties and may help reduce inflammation in the body. Add foods rich in omega-3s to your meal, such as:

    - Fatty fish (salmon, mackerel, sardines)
    - Flaxseeds and flaxseed oil
    - Chia seeds
    - Walnuts

5. **Avoid Trigger Foods:** Identify and avoid foods that trigger symptoms or exacerbate inflammation in your digestive tract. Common trigger foods in Crohn's disease include:

    - Spicy foods
    - High-fiber foods (raw vegetables, whole grains)
    - Dairy products (if lactose intolerant)

- Fatty or fried foods
- Caffeine and alcohol

6. **Small, Frequent Meals:** Eating smaller, more frequent meals throughout the day can help prevent overwhelming your digestive system and minimize symptoms like bloating and discomfort.

7. **Nutrient-Dense Foods:** Focus on consuming nutrient-dense foods to support overall health and optimize nutrient absorption. Add varieties of colorful fruits, vegetables, lean proteins, and whole grains in your diet.

Carefully Selected Food Diet
1. Banana Oatmeal Smoothie

Ingredients

- *1 ripe banana*
- *1/2 cup rolled oats*
- *1 cup almond milk*
- *1 tablespoon honey or maple syrup (optional)*
- *Dash of cinnamon*

Preparation

1. Peel the banana and break it into chunks.
2. Combine banana chunks, rolled oats, almond milk, honey or maple syrup (if using), and cinnamon in a blender.
3. Blend until smooth.
4. If desired, add ice cubes and blend again until smooth.

2. Mashed Sweet Potatoes

Ingredients

- *2 medium sweet potatoes*

- *2 tablespoons butter or olive oil*
- *Salt and pepper to taste*

Preparation

1. Peel the sweet potatoes and cut them into chunks.
2. Place the sweet potato chunks in a pot of boiling water and cook until tender, about 15-20 minutes.
3. Drain the cooked sweet potatoes and return them to the pot.
4. Add butter or olive oil to the pot and mash the sweet potatoes until smooth.
5. Season with salt and pepper to taste.

3. Chicken and Rice Soup

Ingredients

- *2 boneless, skinless chicken breasts*
- *4 cups chicken broth*
- *1 cup cooked rice*

- *2 carrots, chopped*
- *2 celery stalks, chopped*
- *Salt and pepper to taste*

Preparation

1. In a large pot, bring the chicken broth to a simmer.
2. Add the chicken breasts to the pot and simmer until cooked through, about 15-20 minutes.
3. Remove the chicken breasts from the pot and shred them using two forks.
4. Return the shredded chicken to the pot.
5. Add the cooked rice, chopped carrots, and chopped celery to the pot.
6. Simmer the soup until the vegetables are tender, about 10-15 minutes.
7. Season with salt and pepper to taste before serving.

4. Scrambled Eggs with Spinach

Ingredients

- *4 eggs*
- *1 cup fresh spinach, chopped*
- *1 tablespoon olive oil*
- *Salt and pepper to taste*

Preparation

1. In a bowl, whisk together the eggs until well beaten.
2. Heat the olive oil in a skillet over medium heat.
3. Add the chopped spinach to the skillet and sauté until wilted.
4. Pour the beaten eggs into the skillet with the spinach.
5. Cook, stirring occasionally, until the eggs are scrambled and fully cooked.

6. Season with salt and pepper to taste before serving.

5. Baked Salmon with Lemon and Herbs

Ingredients

- *4 salmon fillets*
- *2 tablespoons olive oil*
- *1 lemon, sliced*
- *2 cloves garlic, minced*
- *1 teaspoon dried thyme*
- *Salt and pepper to taste*

Preparation

1. Preheat the oven to 375°F (190°C).
2. Place the salmon fillets on a baking sheet lined with parchment paper.
3. Drizzle olive oil over the salmon fillets and season with minced garlic, dried thyme, salt, and pepper.

4. Place lemon slices on top of each salmon fillet.
5. Bake in the preheated oven for 12-15 minutes, or until the salmon is cooked through and flakes easily with a fork.

6. **Quinoa Salad with Cucumber and Tomato**

Ingredients

- *1 cup quinoa, rinsed*
- *2 cups water or vegetable broth*
- *1 cucumber, diced*
- *1 cup cherry tomatoes, halved*
- *1/4 cup chopped fresh parsley*
- *2 tablespoons olive oil*
- *2 tablespoons lemon juice*
- *Salt and pepper to taste*

Preparation

1. In a saucepan, combine the quinoa and water or vegetable broth. Bring to a boil, then reduce heat to low, cover, and simmer for 15-20 minutes, or until the quinoa is cooked and the liquid is absorbed.
2. Fluff the cooked quinoa with a fork and transfer it to a large bowl.
3. Add the diced cucumber, halved cherry tomatoes, and chopped parsley to the bowl with the quinoa.
4. Drizzle olive oil and lemon juice over the salad, then toss to combine.
5. Season with salt and pepper to taste before serving.

7. **Steamed Vegetables with Garlic Butter**

Ingredients

- *Assorted vegetables (e.g., broccoli, cauliflower, carrots), chopped*
- *2 tablespoons butter*

- *2 cloves garlic, minced*
- *Salt and pepper to taste*

Preparation

1. Steam the chopped vegetables until tender, either using a steamer basket or by boiling them in a pot of water.
2. In a small saucepan, melt the butter over low heat.
3. Add minced garlic to the melted butter and cook for 1-2 minutes, until fragrant.
4. Drizzle the garlic butter over the steamed vegetables.
5. Season with salt and pepper to taste before serving.

8. **Turkey and Vegetable Stir-Fry**

Ingredients

- *1 lb turkey breast, thinly sliced*

- *2 cups mixed vegetables (e.g., bell peppers, snap peas, mushrooms), sliced*
- *2 tablespoons soy sauce*
- *1 tablespoon olive oil*
- *2 cloves garlic, minced*
- *1 teaspoon grated ginger*
- *Cooked rice or quinoa for serving*

Preparation

1. Heat olive oil in a large skillet or wok over medium-high heat.

2. Add minced garlic and grated ginger to the skillet, and stir-fry for 1 minute until fragrant.

3. Add thinly sliced turkey breast to the skillet and cook until browned and cooked through.

4. Add sliced mixed vegetables to the skillet and stir-fry until tender-crisp.

5. Pour soy sauce over the turkey and vegetable mixture, and stir to combine.

6. Serve the turkey and vegetable stir-fry over cooked rice or quinoa.

9. **Greek Yogurt Parfait with Berries and Granola**

Ingredients

- *1 cup Greek yogurt*
- *1/2 cup mixed berries (e.g., strawberries, blueberries, raspberries)*
- *1/4 cup granola*
- *Honey or maple syrup (optional)*

Preparation

1. In a serving glass or bowl, layer Greek yogurt, mixed berries, and granola.

2. Repeat the layers until the glass or bowl is filled.

3. Drizzle honey or maple syrup over the top if desired.

4. Serve immediately as a healthy breakfast or snack option.

10. Spinach and Feta Stuffed Chicken Breast

Ingredients

- *4 boneless, skinless chicken breasts*
- *2 cups fresh spinach leaves*
- *1/2 cup crumbled feta cheese*
- *2 cloves garlic, minced*
- *1 tablespoon olive oil*
- *Salt and pepper to taste*

Preparation

1. Preheat the oven to 375°F (190°C).

2. In a skillet, heat olive oil over medium heat. Add minced garlic and cook until fragrant.

3. Add fresh spinach leaves to the skillet and cook until wilted. Remove from heat and let cool slightly.

4. Butterfly each chicken breast by slicing horizontally through the middle, leaving one edge intact, to create a pocket.

5. Stuff each chicken breast with cooked spinach and crumbled feta cheese.

6. Season the stuffed chicken breasts with salt and pepper.

7. Place the stuffed chicken breasts in a baking dish and bake in the preheated oven for 25-30 minutes, or until the chicken is cooked through.

11. **Vegetable Lentil Soup**

Ingredients

- *1 cup green lentils, rinsed*
- *4 cups vegetable broth*
- *1 onion, diced*
- *2 carrots, diced*
- *2 celery stalks, diced*
- *2 cloves garlic, minced*
- *1 teaspoon ground cumin*
- *1 teaspoon ground turmeric*
- *Salt and pepper to taste*
- *Fresh parsley for garnish*

Preparation

1. In a large pot, combine green lentils and vegetable broth. Bring to a boil, then reduce heat to low, cover, and simmer for 20-25 minutes, or until the lentils are tender.

2. In a separate skillet, heat olive oil over medium heat. Add diced onion, carrots, and celery, and cook until softened.

3. Add minced garlic, ground cumin, and ground turmeric to the skillet, and cook for an additional 1-2 minutes.

4. Transfer the cooked vegetables to the pot with the lentils and broth.

5. Season the soup with salt and pepper to taste.

6. Serve hot, garnished with fresh parsley.

12. **Roasted Vegetable Quinoa Bowl**

Ingredients

- *1 cup quinoa, rinsed*
- *2 cups water or vegetable broth*
- *2 cups mixed vegetables (e.g., bell peppers, zucchini, cherry tomatoes), chopped*
- *2 tablespoons olive oil*

- *1 teaspoon dried Italian seasoning*
- *Salt and pepper to taste*
- *Feta cheese for garnish (optional)*

<u>Preparation</u>

1. Preheat the oven to 400°F (200°C).

2. In a saucepan, combine quinoa and water or vegetable broth. Bring to a boil, then reduce heat to low, cover, and simmer for 15-20 minutes, or until the quinoa is cooked and the liquid is absorbed.

3. While the quinoa is cooking, spread chopped mixed vegetables on a baking sheet lined with parchment paper.

4. Drizzle olive oil over the vegetables and sprinkle with dried Italian seasoning, salt, and pepper.

5. Roast the vegetables in the preheated oven for 20-25 minutes, or until tender and slightly caramelized.

6. To assemble the quinoa bowls, divide cooked quinoa among serving bowls and top with roasted vegetables.

7. Garnish with crumbled feta cheese if desired before serving.

13. **Turkey and Vegetable Skewers**

Ingredients

- *1 lb turkey breast, cut into cubes*
- *2 bell peppers, cut into chunks*
- *1 zucchini, sliced*
- *1 red onion, cut into chunks*
- *8-10 cherry tomatoes*
- *2 tablespoons olive oil*

- *1 tablespoon balsamic vinegar*
- *1 teaspoon dried oregano*
- *Salt and pepper to taste*

Preparation

1. Preheat the grill to medium-high heat.
2. In a bowl, whisk together olive oil, balsamic vinegar, dried oregano, salt, and pepper to make the marinade.
3. Thread turkey cubes, bell pepper chunks, zucchini slices, red onion chunks, and cherry tomatoes onto skewers, alternating between ingredients.
4. Brush the skewers with the prepared marinade.
5. Grill the skewers for 10-12 minutes, turning occasionally, until the turkey is cooked through and the vegetables are tender.

6. Serve hot as a delicious and healthy meal option.

14. Mediterranean Chickpea Salad

Ingredients

- 1 can (15 oz) chickpeas, drained and rinsed
- 1 cucumber, diced
- 1 cup cherry tomatoes, halved
- 1/4 cup Kalamata olives, pitted and halved
- 1/4 cup crumbled feta cheese
- 2 tablespoons chopped fresh parsley
- 2 tablespoons olive oil
- 1 tablespoon lemon juice
- 1 teaspoon dried oregano
- Salt and pepper to taste

Preparation

1. In a large bowl, combine chickpeas, diced cucumber, halved cherry tomatoes, halved Kalamata olives, crumbled feta cheese, and chopped fresh parsley.

2. In a small bowl, whisk together olive oil, lemon juice, dried oregano, salt, and pepper to make the dressing.

3. Pour the dressing over the chickpea salad and toss to combine.

4. Serve chilled as a refreshing and nutritious salad option.

15. Honey Garlic Shrimp Stir-Fry

Ingredients

- *1 lb shrimp, peeled and deveined*

- *2 cups mixed vegetables (e.g., bell peppers, broccoli, snap peas), sliced*

- *3 cloves garlic, minced*

- *2 tablespoons honey*
- *1 tablespoon soy sauce*
- *1 tablespoon olive oil*
- *Sesame seeds for garnish*
- *Cooked rice or quinoa for serving*

Preparation

1. In a small bowl, whisk together minced garlic, honey, and soy sauce to make the sauce.//
2. Heat olive oil in a large skillet or wok over medium-high heat.
3. Add shrimp to the skillet and cook until pink and opaque.
4. Add sliced mixed vegetables to the skillet and stir-fry until tender-crisp.

5. Pour the prepared sauce over the shrimp and vegetables, and toss to coat evenly.

6. Cook for an additional 1-2 minutes, until the sauce thickens slightly.

7. Serve the honey garlic shrimp stir-fry over cooked rice or quinoa, garnished with sesame seeds.

16. Stuffed Bell Peppers with Turkey and Quinoa

Ingredients

- *4 large bell peppers*
- *1 lb ground turkey*
- *1 cup cooked quinoa*
- *1 cup tomato sauce*
- *1 onion, diced*
- *2 cloves garlic, minced*
- *1 teaspoon dried Italian seasoning*

- *Salt and pepper to taste*

- *Shredded mozzarella cheese for topping*

Preparation

1. Preheat the oven to 375°F (190°C).

2. Cut the tops off the bell peppers and remove the seeds and membranes from the inside.

3. In a skillet, cook ground turkey over medium heat until browned and cooked through. Drain excess fat if needed.

4. Add diced onion and minced garlic to the skillet with the cooked turkey, and cook until softened.

5. Stir in cooked quinoa, tomato sauce, dried Italian seasoning, salt, and pepper, and cook for an additional 2-3 minutes.

6. Spoon the turkey and quinoa mixture into the hollowed-out bell peppers.

7. Place the stuffed bell peppers in a baking dish and cover with foil.

8. Bake in the preheated oven for 25-30 minutes, or until the peppers are tender.

9. Remove the foil and sprinkle shredded mozzarella cheese over the tops of the stuffed peppers.

10. Return to the oven and bake for an additional 5 minutes, or until the cheese is melted and bubbly.

17. **Vegetarian Lentil Curry**

Ingredients

- *1 cup green lentils, rinsed*
- *4 cups vegetable broth*
- *1 onion, diced*

- *2 cloves garlic, minced*
- *1 tablespoon grated ginger*
- *1 tablespoon curry powder*
- *1 teaspoon ground cumin*
- *1 teaspoon ground turmeric*
- *1 can (14 oz) diced tomatoes*
- *1 can (14 oz) coconut milk*
- *Salt and pepper to taste*
- *Fresh cilantro for garnish*

Preparation

1. In a large pot, combine green lentils and vegetable broth. Bring to a boil, then reduce heat to low, cover, and simmer for 20-25 minutes, or until the lentils are tender.

2. In a separate skillet, heat olive oil over medium heat. Add diced onion and cook until softened.

3. Add minced garlic, grated ginger, curry powder, ground cumin, and ground turmeric to the skillet, and cook for an additional 1-2 minutes.

4. Stir in diced tomatoes and coconut milk, and bring to a simmer.

5. Add the cooked lentils to the skillet with the curry sauce, and stir to combine.

6. Season with salt and pepper to taste.

7. Simmer the vegetarian lentil curry for an additional 5-10 minutes to allow the flavors to meld.

8. Serve hot, garnished with fresh cilantro.

18. **Baked Chicken Meatballs**

Ingredients

- *1 lb ground chicken*
- *1/2 cup breadcrumbs*
- *1/4 cup grated Parmesan cheese*
- *1 egg*
- *2 cloves garlic, minced*
- *2 tablespoons chopped fresh parsley*
- *1 teaspoon dried oregano*
- *Salt and pepper to taste*

Preparation

1. Preheat the oven to 400°F (200°C). Line a baking sheet with parchment paper.
2. In a large bowl, combine ground chicken, breadcrumbs, grated Parmesan cheese, egg, minced garlic, chopped fresh parsley, dried oregano, salt, and pepper.

3. Mix until well combined, then shape the mixture into meatballs using your hands.
4. Place the chicken meatballs on the prepared baking sheet.
5. Bake in the preheated oven for 20-25 minutes, or until the meatballs are cooked through and golden brown.
6. Serve hot with your favorite sauce or as a protein-rich addition to salads, pastas, or grain bowls.

19. **Vegetable Frittata**

Ingredients

- *8 large eggs*
- *1 cup mixed vegetables (e.g., bell peppers, spinach, onions), chopped*
- *1/2 cup shredded cheese (e.g., cheddar, mozzarella)*
- *2 tablespoons olive oil*

- *Salt and pepper to taste*

Preparation

1. Preheat the oven to 350°F (175°C).

2. In a bowl, whisk together eggs, salt, and pepper until well beaten.

3. Heat olive oil in an oven-safe skillet over medium heat.

4. Add chopped mixed vegetables to the skillet and cook until softened.

5. Pour the beaten eggs over the cooked vegetables in the skillet, then sprinkle shredded cheese on top.

6. Cook on the stovetop for 3-4 minutes, or until the edges of the frittata begin to set.

7. Transfer the skillet to the preheated oven and bake for 10-12 minutes, or until the frittata is set and golden brown.

8. Remove from the oven and let cool slightly before slicing into wedges.

9. Serve warm or at room temperature as a nutritious and satisfying meal option.

20. Vegetable Stir-Fried Rice

Ingredients

- *2 cups cooked rice (preferably cooled)*
- *2 cups mixed vegetables (e.g., carrots, peas, corn)*
- *2 tablespoons soy sauce*
- *1 tablespoon sesame oil*
- *2 cloves garlic, minced*
- *2 green onions, sliced*
- *2 eggs, beaten*
- Salt and pepper to taste

Preparation

1. Heat sesame oil in a large skillet or wok over medium-high heat.
2. Add minced garlic to the skillet and stir-fry for 1 minute until fragrant.
3. Add mixed vegetables to the skillet and stir-fry until tender-crisp.
4. Push the vegetables to one side of the skillet, then pour beaten eggs into the empty space.
5. Scramble the eggs until cooked, then mix them with the cooked vegetables.
6. Add cooked rice to the skillet, breaking up any clumps, and stir-fry until heated through.
7. Drizzle soy sauce over the rice and vegetable mixture, and toss to combine.
8. Season with salt and pepper to taste, then garnish with sliced green onions before serving.

9. Serve hot as a delicious and filling meal option.

21. Salmon and Asparagus Foil Packets

Ingredients

- *4 salmon fillets*
- *1 lb asparagus spears, trimmed*
- *2 tablespoons olive oil*
- *2 cloves garlic, minced*
- *1 lemon, thinly sliced*
- *Salt and pepper to taste*
- *Fresh dill for garnish*

Preparation

1. Preheat the oven to 375°F (190°C).
2. Place each salmon fillet on a large piece of aluminum foil.

3. Arrange asparagus spears around each salmon fillet.

4. Drizzle olive oil over the salmon and asparagus, then sprinkle minced garlic on top.

5. Season with salt and pepper to taste, then place lemon slices on top of each salmon fillet.

6. Fold the edges of the aluminum foil to create sealed packets.

7. Place the foil packets on a baking sheet and bake in the preheated oven for 15-20 minutes, or until the salmon is cooked through and the asparagus is tender.

8. Carefully open the foil packets, garnish with fresh dill, and serve hot.

22. **Greek Chicken Souvlaki with Tzatziki Sauce**

Ingredients

- 1 lb chicken breast, cut into cubes
- 1/4 cup olive oil
- 2 tablespoons lemon juice
- 2 cloves garlic, minced
- 1 teaspoon dried oregano
- Salt and pepper to taste
- Wooden skewers, soaked in water
- Tzatziki sauce for serving

Preparation

1. In a bowl, whisk together olive oil, lemon juice, minced garlic, dried oregano, salt, and pepper to make the marinade.

2. Add chicken cubes to the marinade and toss to coat evenly. Cover and refrigerate for at least 30 minutes, or up to 4 hours.

3. Preheat the grill to medium-high heat.

4. Thread marinated chicken cubes onto soaked wooden skewers.

5. Grill the chicken skewers for 8-10 minutes, turning occasionally, until cooked through and slightly charred.

6. Serve hot with tzatziki sauce for dipping and your choice of sides.

23. Spaghetti Squash with Marinara Sauce:
Ingredients

- *1 spaghetti squash*
- *2 cups marinara sauce (store-bought or homemade)*
- *2 tablespoons olive oil*
- *2 cloves garlic, minced*
- *Salt and pepper to taste*

- *Fresh basil for garnish*

Preparation

1. Preheat the oven to 400°F (200°C).

2. Cut the spaghetti squash in half lengthwise and scoop out the seeds.

3. Drizzle olive oil over the cut sides of the spaghetti squash, then season with minced garlic, salt, and pepper.

4. Place the squash halves, cut side down, on a baking sheet lined with parchment paper.

5. Roast in the preheated oven for 30-40 minutes, or until the squash is tender and the flesh can be easily scraped into strands with a fork.

6. While the squash is roasting, heat marinara sauce in a saucepan over medium heat until heated through.

7. Once the spaghetti squash is cooked, use a fork to scrape the flesh into strands.

8. Serve the spaghetti squash topped with marinara sauce and garnished with fresh basil.

24. **Turkey and Vegetable Chili:**

Ingredients

- *1 lb ground turkey*

- *1 onion, diced*

- *2 cloves garlic, minced*

- *2 bell peppers, diced*

- *2 carrots, diced*

- *1 zucchini, diced*

- *1 can (15 oz) diced tomatoes*

- *1 can (15 oz) kidney beans, drained and rinsed*

- *1 cup vegetable broth*

- *2 tablespoons chili powder*
- *1 teaspoon ground cumin*
- *Salt and pepper to taste*
- *Fresh cilantro for garnish*

Preparation

1. In a large pot, cook ground turkey over medium heat until browned and cooked through. Drain excess fat if needed.

2. Add diced onion and minced garlic to the pot with the cooked turkey, and cook until softened.

3. Add diced bell peppers, carrots, and zucchini to the pot, and cook until slightly softened.

4. Stir in diced tomatoes, kidney beans, vegetable broth, chili powder, ground cumin, salt, and pepper.

5. Bring the chili to a simmer and cook for 20-25 minutes, stirring occasionally, until the vegetables are tender and the flavors are well combined.

6. Serve hot, garnished with fresh cilantro.

25. Quinoa Stuffed Bell Peppers:

Ingredients

- *4 large bell peppers*
- *1 cup quinoa, rinsed*
- *2 cups vegetable broth*
- *1 onion, diced*
- *2 cloves garlic, minced*
- *1 can (15 oz) black beans, drained and rinsed*
- *1 can (15 oz) diced tomatoes*
- *1 teaspoon chili powder*
- *1 teaspoon ground cumin*

- *Salt and pepper to taste*

- *Shredded cheddar cheese for topping*

Preparation

1. Preheat the oven to 375°F (190°C).

2. Cut the tops off the bell peppers and remove the seeds and membranes from the inside.

3. In a saucepan, combine quinoa and vegetable broth. Bring to a boil, then reduce heat to low, cover, and simmer for 15-20 minutes, or until the quinoa is cooked and the liquid is absorbed.

4. In a skillet, heat olive oil over medium heat. Add diced onion and cook until softened.

5. Add minced garlic, black beans, diced tomatoes, chili powder, ground cumin, salt,

and pepper to the skillet, and cook for an additional 2-3 minutes.

6. Stir cooked quinoa into the skillet with the bean and tomato mixture, and mix until well combined.

7. Spoon the quinoa mixture into the hollowed-out bell peppers.

8. Place the stuffed bell peppers in a baking dish and cover with foil.

9. Bake in the preheated oven for 25-30 minutes, or until the peppers are tender.

10. Remove the foil and sprinkle shredded cheddar cheese over the tops of the stuffed peppers.

11. Return to the oven and bake for an additional 5 minutes, or until the cheese is melted and bubbly.

Some Key Facts About Crohn's Disease

- Crohn's disease is a long-term inflammatory disorder that mainly impacts the gastrointestinal tract.

- It can cause symptoms such as abdominal pain, diarrhea, weight loss, fatigue, and malnutrition.

- The precise cause of Crohn's disease remains unclear, though it is thought to result from a combination of genetic, environmental, and immune system factors.

- Crohn's disease can affect people of any age, but it's most commonly diagnosed in adolescents and young adults.

- There is currently no cure for Crohn's disease, but various treatments, including medications, lifestyle changes, and sometimes surgery, can help manage symptoms and improve quality of life.

- Complications of Crohn's disease may include intestinal strictures, fistulas, abscesses, nutritional deficiencies, and an increased risk of colorectal cancer.

- Treatment plans for Crohn's disease are individualized based on the severity of symptoms, disease location, and other factors, and may require ongoing monitoring and adjustments.

- Living with Crohn's disease can be challenging, but with proper management and support, many people with the condition are able to lead active and fulfilling lives.

Medical Advice and Tips

1. Follow your treatment plan diligently, including taking medications as prescribed and attending regular check-ups with your healthcare provider.

2. Maintain a healthy diet that is tailored to your individual needs and avoids trigger foods that worsen your symptoms.

3. Stay hydrated by drinking plenty of fluids, especially water, throughout the day to help prevent dehydration, which can worsen symptoms.

4. Manage stress effectively through techniques such as relaxation exercises, mindfulness meditation, deep breathing, or engaging in hobbies and activities you enjoy.

5. Get regular exercise to promote overall physical and mental well-being. Choose

activities that you enjoy and can comfortably incorporate into your daily routine.

6. Practice good hygiene, especially when it comes to food preparation and handwashing, to reduce the risk of infections and other complications.

7. Keep track of your symptoms and any changes in your condition, and communicate openly with your healthcare team about your concerns or questions.

8. Seek support from friends, family members, or support groups who understand what you're going through and can provide encouragement, empathy, and practical advice.

9. Be proactive in managing your healthcare by educating yourself about Crohn's disease, staying informed about new treatments and

research developments, and advocating for your needs and preferences.

10. Don't hesitate to reach out for help if you're struggling emotionally or mentally. Therapy, counseling, or support groups can provide valuable resources and coping strategies for dealing with the challenges of living with Crohn's disease.

Glossary of Terms

1. **Crohn's Disease**: A chronic inflammatory condition of the gastrointestinal tract, characterized by inflammation that can affect any part of the digestive system.

2. **Inflammatory Bowel Disease (IBD)**: A group of chronic inflammatory conditions of the gastrointestinal tract, including Crohn's disease and ulcerative colitis.

3. **Gastrointestinal Tract (GI Tract)**: The series of organs that make up the digestive system, including the mouth, esophagus, stomach, small intestine, large intestine (colon), rectum, and anus.

4. **Inflammation**: The body's response to injury, infection, or irritation, characterized by redness, swelling, heat, and pain. In Crohn's

disease, inflammation occurs in the gastrointestinal tract.

5. **Remission**: A period of time when symptoms of Crohn's disease are reduced or absent, and the condition is less active.

6. **Flare-up**: A sudden worsening of symptoms of Crohn's disease, often characterized by increased inflammation and gastrointestinal symptoms such as abdominal pain and diarrhea.

7. **Immune System**: The body's defense system against infection and disease, consisting of specialized cells and proteins that work together to identify and destroy foreign invaders.

8. **Fistula**: An abnormal connection or passageway that forms between two organs or tissues that are not normally connected, often

occurring in Crohn's disease between different parts of the intestine or between the intestine and other organs.

9. **Stricture**: Abnormal narrowing of a passage or tube in the body, such as the intestines, due to scar tissue or inflammation, which can cause blockages and obstruct the flow of fluids or food.

10. **Biopsy**: A procedure in which a small sample of tissue is removed from the body for examination under a microscope, often used to diagnose Crohn's disease and evaluate inflammation or abnormalities in the gastrointestinal tract.

11. **Colonoscopy**: A procedure in which a flexible tube with a camera is inserted into the rectum and advanced through the colon to examine the lining of the colon and rectum for signs of inflammation, ulcers, or other abnormalities.

12. **MRI Enterography**: A specialized imaging technique that uses magnetic resonance imaging (MRI) to visualize the small intestine and detect inflammation or other abnormalities, often used to evaluate Crohn's disease.

13. **Nutrition Therapy**: Dietary interventions aimed at managing symptoms and improving nutritional status in individuals with Crohn's disease, including enteral nutrition (nutrition through a feeding tube) or parenteral nutrition (nutrition through an intravenous line).

14. **Lifestyle Modifications**: Changes in daily habits and activities, such as diet, exercise, stress management, and smoking cessation, aimed at reducing symptoms and improving overall well-being in individuals with Crohn's disease.

15. **Surgery**: A treatment option for severe or complicated cases of Crohn's disease that involves removing damaged portions of the intestine, repairing fistulas or strictures, or addressing complications such as abscesses or bowel obstructions.

www.ingramcontent.com/pod-product-compliance
Lightning Source LLC
Chambersburg PA
CBHW050234230526
45470CB00005B/1946